C000126528

Resista

exercise

COMPLETE GUIDE TO KEEP YOU FIT

COPYRIGHT@2019

By

PT. ALEX UHUN

Table of Contents

ways that to progress your exercises before adding weights, or are simply on the look for an excellent exercise tool that is versatile and instantly adds resistance on the go, its value finance in some bands.

Chapter 2

What do resistance bands do?

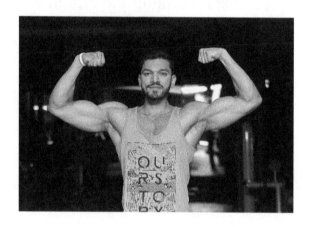

A resistance band will specifically what the name suggests: it adds resistance to Associate in nursing exercise. This additional resistance helps strengthen your muscles and pushes you to figure a bit more durable.

Resistance bands have variety of advantages. Additionally to their ability to assist you strengthen muscles teams, they're additionally cheap, moveable and accessible.

Tone and strengthen

As resistance bands stretch, they produce inflated tension in your muscles and cause them to contract. The additional you stretch the band, the additional intense the resistance gets, and therefore the tougher the exercise becomes. you'll be able to additionally produce additional resistance by holding the resistance band in a very manner will increase tension – like transferal your hands nearer along once doing arm moves, for instance.

Add help, not simply resistance

Resistance bands may assist your progress with troublesome exercises. As an example, for those needing to restore at pull-ups, merely attach the resistance band to the bar Associate in Nursing either underneath your knee or foot to figure your high to an unassisted version. As you perform the pull-up with the band, your weight is supported by the band, creating the exercise a lot of accessible.

Great for stretching

These elastic bands are an incredible addition to your stretching routine, particularly if you lack flexibility and quality. A resistance band allows you to extend vary of motion and deepen the stretch as you gently move the band either away or towards your body.

Lightweight and moveable

These bands build the proper companion to those desirous to exercise once traveling. They extraordinarily light-weight and might simply be stashed in your luggage or baggage.

Resistance bands work your muscles like weights do – your muscles contract to come up with force to stabilize and management the specified movement. However, in contrast to weights, resistance bands don't place confidence in gravity to produce the resistance. This implies that the body will move and expand vary of motion in sure exercises (e.g. elevate the arms higher during a handgun lift).

Resistance bands square measure cheap, cost accounting anyplace between $5-10. Simply bear in mind that the thicker the band, the additional resistance can it'll} have that the more durable the exercises will become. Choose a range pack thus you mostly have varied resistances to decide on from.

Chapter 3

Looped Resistance Band

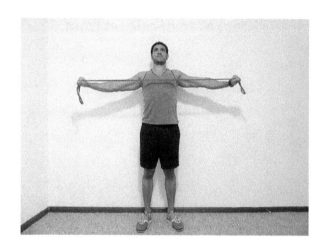

Band Pull Apart

Targets: Chest, triceps, rhomboids
(upper back)

Guide:

1. Stand along with your feet
shoulder-width apart and head
facing forward

2. Hold a resistance band before
of you along with your arms
extended straight out. There
ought to be 4-6 inches of band
left at the ends wherever your
grip stops Pull the band apart
by transferal your shoulder
blades along so the band
touches your chest

3. Slowly come back to the beginning position by transferal your arms back off before you at eye level. This move ought to be done slowly and in restraint. Repeat for 8-10 reps
4. You'll be able to use a medical care band for this exercise, if strength bands are too troublesome.

Chapter 4

Upright Row

Targets: Shoulders

Guide:

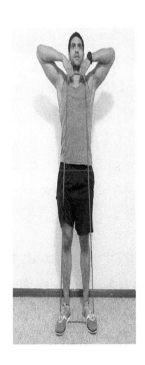

1. Stand with the band below your feet, shoulder-width apart. Shoulders ought to be back, spine straight and head facing forward

2. Hold the highest of the band with a pronated (overhand) grip, hands close and arms straight down ahead of your body. This can be the beginning position

3. Raise your hands towards toward ceiling, raising them to concerning chin height, whereas keeping the hands

about to the body. Your elbows
ought to purpose to your sides
and your forearms parallel to
the ground

4. Return the bands back to the
beginning position

5. Repeat for 8-10 reps.

Chapter 5

Bicep Curl

Targets: striated muscle

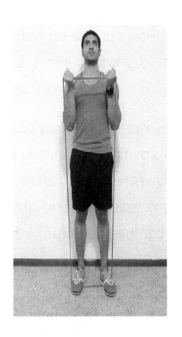

How to: rise up tall with feet shoulder-width apart, band whorled below your feet

Grab the highest of the band employing a supinated (underhand) grip with hands outside of hips and arms extended straight down. This can be the beginning position

Raise the band to concerning chin height along with your arms bent into a curl and elbows inform to the ground

(c). Then, bring the band backtrack to the beginning position with management. That's one rep

(d). Repeat for 8-10 reps.

For AN intense pump: Set a timer for thirty seconds and do as several reps as potential. You'll be able to sacrifice full vary of motion towards the top if you get tired, in favor of flushing a lot of blood to the striated muscle.

Chapter 6

Push-Up with Band

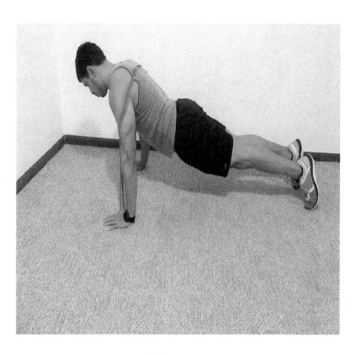

Targets: Chest, triceps, shoulders

Guide:

1. Lay flat on your abdomen together with your legs straight behind you and toes tucked.

2. Place the resistance band behind you thus it's lying across your mid-back.

3. Then, hold the band together with your hands in order that

every thumb is within every finish of the loop.

4. Your hands shoulder-width apart, and arms area unit at your sides together with your elbows bent

5. Do a push-up against the band to full extension, keeping your butt back in an exceedingly line.

6. . Then, slowly bring your body backpedal to the bottom

7. Repeat for 8-10 reps

Chapter 7

Mini Band- Lateral Band Walk

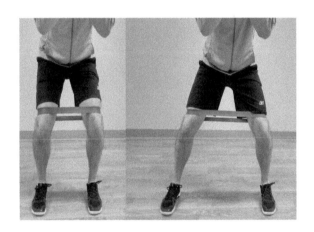

Targets: Hips, gluts, quadriceps, hamstrings

GUIDE:

1. Place the resistance band around your ankles and acquire into a squat position along with

your thighs parallel to the bottom and feet slightly wider than hip-distance apart

2. Exit to the left (laterally) against the band, remaining within the squat position along with your hands ahead you in associate athletic stance

3. Alternate sides and step to your right against the band

4. Exit 5 times on all sides

5. To extend the issue of this exercise and acquire a pleasant shoulder stretch, too, do identical exercise along with your hands and arms extended overhead

6. Repeat for 8-10 reps.

Chapter 8

Plank Jack

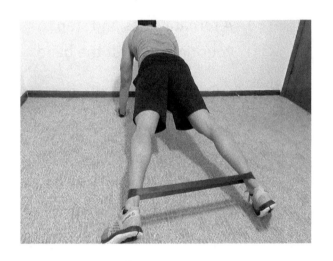

Targets: Abs, gluts

1. Place the resistance band
    around your ankles and find
    into push-up position together
    with your hands shoulder-
    width apart, and hips upraised
    and aligned together with your
    back

2. Jack each legs bent on your sides till you're feeling a stretch in your core and glutes

3. Bring your legs back to the beginning position. This move ought to be done quickly to stay tension within the core in the slightest degree times. Keep core tight throughout the motion

4. Do 8-10 reps.

Chapter 9

Lying skeletal muscle Bridge with motility

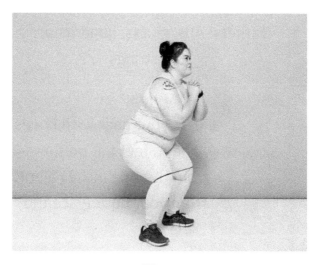

Targets: Abs, glutes, quadriceps, hamstrings

Guide:

1. Lie on your back with knees bent, feet flat on the ground, some inches aloof from your butt. Place the

resistance band slightly
below knees
2. Press into a bridge by
raising your hips and butt
off the ground pushing
them as high as attainable
towards ceiling. Keep your
shoulders anchored to the
ground, so that they
produce a diagonal line to
your knees
3. Now, push against the band
to separate your legs till
you're feeling a stretch in
your glutes
4. come legs back to center
then bring backpedal to
ground
5. Repeat for 8-10 reps.

Chapter 10

Resistance Band Front Raise

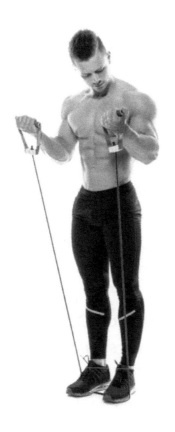

Targets: Front delts

1. Stand on prime of the
resistance band along with
your feet shoulder-width apart
whereas holding one handle in
every hand with AN overhand
grip
2. Keeping your shoulders back
and spine straight, bring each
handles up to eye level by
extending shoulders straight
intent on the edges.
3. Slowly bring the handles
backtrack with management
4. Repeat for 8-10 reps.

Chapter 11

Resistance Band Bent-Over

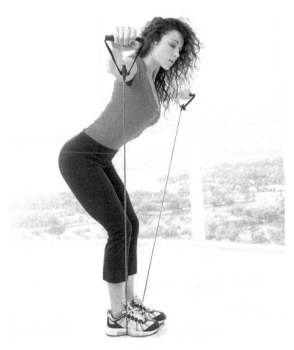

Targets: Deltoids

Guide:

1. Stand along with your feet hip-distance apart on high of the resistance band, hinging slightly forward. Keep your gaze on the bottom. Hold bands with a neutral (palms facing every other) grip and arms straight at your sides

2. Raise each arms towards the ceiling till your arms reach shoulder height
3. Bring the bands backtrack to the beginning position. Elbows is slightly bent throughout this motion
4. Repeat for 8-10 reps.

Chapter 12

Squat to Press

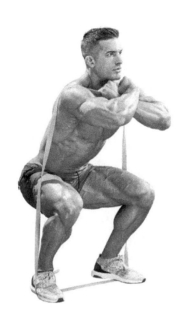

Targets: Full Body

Guide:

1. Stand on high of the resistance band with feet hip-distance apart. Hold the handles with associate overhand grip and your arms at shoulder-level, like you're near to press them up overhead

2. Drop into a squat therefore your knees area unit nearly directly over your toes and thighs area unit parallel to the ground. make certain to stay your hands by your shoulders

3. Slowly return up to standing, pressing the handles up overhead till your arms area unit totally extended

4. Bring your arms back to shoulder-height

5. Repeat the exercise in one fluid
   motion: Squat, then press up
6. Do 8-10 reps.